Sjogren's Syndrome

A Beginner's 3-Step Guide for Women on Managing the Condition Through Diet, With Sample Recipes and a 7-Day Meal Plan

mf

Disclaimer

By reading this disclaimer, you are accepting the terms of the disclaimer in full. If you disagree with this disclaimer, please do not read the guide.

All of the content within this guide is provided for informational and educational purposes only, and should not be accepted as independent medical or other professional advice. The author is not a doctor, physician, nurse, mental health provider, or registered nutritionist/dietician. Therefore, using and reading this guide does not establish any form of a physician-patient relationship.

Always consult with a physician or another qualified health provider with any issues or questions you might have regarding any sort of medical condition. Do not ever disregard any qualified professional medical advice or delay seeking that advice because of anything you have read in this guide. The information in this guide is not intended to be any sort of medical advice and should not be used in lieu of any medical advice by a licensed and qualified medical professional.

The information in this guide has been compiled from a variety of known sources. However, the author cannot attest to or guarantee the accuracy of each source and thus should not be held liable for any errors or omissions.

Table of Contents

Introduction

Life with Sjogren's Syndrome often feels like navigating an uphill terrain without a clear map. It's an autoimmune disorder that doesn't always get the attention it deserves, yet its effects can seep into nearly every corner of someone's daily life. From the outside, it might just seem like dry eyes or fatigue, but for those living with it, this condition often goes far beyond the surface.

Sjogren's Syndrome is a chronic condition where the immune system mistakenly attacks the glands that produce moisture, leading to a range of symptoms. However, it can often take time to receive a proper diagnosis.

Its symptoms can overlap with other conditions, and the unpredictability can leave people feeling isolated or frustrated. Understanding the condition becomes vital—not just for those diagnosed but for their loved ones, too. Knowledge opens the door to better management, empathy, and support.

In this guide, we will talk about the following;

- Understanding Sjogren's Syndrome
- Diagnosing Sjogren's Syndrome
- Women and Sjogren's Syndrome
- Challenges in Childbearing and Parenting with Sjogren's Syndrome
- The Connection Between Sjogren's Syndrome and Other Autoimmune Diseases
- Mental Health and Emotional Coping with Sjogren's Syndrome
- Supporting Families and Caregivers
- Managing Sjogren's Syndrome Through Diet
- 3-Step Plan for Implementing This Diet

Living well with Sjogren's Syndrome is about finding ways to adapt, seeking the right care, and building a supportive network. Whether someone is navigating this for themselves or assisting a loved one, this guide offers tools, insights, and a sense of clarity. It's about living with purpose and agency, even when a chronic condition tries to complicate things.

Keep reading to learn more about Sjogren's Syndrome and how to manage its many challenges. By the end, you'll have a better understanding of this condition and how to live well with it. You'll also find helpful tips and resources for supporting yourself or your loved ones along the way.

Understanding Sjogren's Syndrome

Sjogren's Syndrome is a long-term autoimmune disease that mainly affects the body's exocrine glands, causing dryness in areas like the mouth and eyes. This systemic condition can affect many other parts of the body, causing a range of symptoms and complications.

The disease is named after Dr. Henrik Sjögren, a Swedish ophthalmologist, who first described its key features in 1933. While cases resembling Sjogren's Syndrome were documented earlier, it was Dr. Sjögren who highlighted the triad of symptoms—dry eyes, dry mouth, and arthritis. His work, based on 19 patients, laid the foundation for distinguishing this condition from other rheumatic diseases.

Dr. Sjögren's observations and mid-20th-century immunology advancements revealed that Sjögren's Syndrome is an autoimmune disorder. The discovery of specific autoantibodies like anti-SSA (Ro) and anti-SSB (La) was a key breakthrough.

The Autoimmune Nature of Sjogren's Syndrome

Sjogren's Syndrome arises when the immune system mistakenly attacks the body's healthy tissues and cells, especially those of the exocrine glands. Normally, the immune system defends the body from harmful invaders like viruses and bacteria. However, in autoimmune diseases like Sjogren's Syndrome, this defense mechanism malfunctions.

The exact cause of this misdirected immune response is not completely understood, but a combination of genetic predisposition, hormonal factors, and environmental triggers is suspected. Women, particularly those aged 40–60, are disproportionately affected, suggesting a link to hormonal influences. Viral infections may also act as triggers, initiating the abnormal immune process that leads to glandular damage.

Symptoms of Sjogren's Syndrome

The symptoms of Sjogren's Syndrome can vary from person to person, and they may also overlap with those of other diseases. The three hallmark signs are dry eyes, dry mouth, and arthritis. Other common symptoms include fatigue, joint pain, and dry skin.

1. *Dry Eyes:* A persistent feeling of grittiness, irritation, or burning in the eyes, often accompanied by redness and sensitivity to light. This can make it uncomfortable

to read, use screens, or even be outside in windy conditions.

2. *Dry Mouth:* A noticeable lack of saliva that can cause difficulty swallowing, speaking, or tasting food. It can also lead to frequent thirst, bad breath, and an increased risk of cavities or gum disease due to reduced saliva's protective effects.

3. *Swelling:* Swelling of the salivary glands, particularly those located behind the jaw and in front of the ears (parotid glands). This swelling may cause discomfort or tenderness and is often more noticeable when eating or drinking.

4. *Joint Pain:* Pain, swelling, and stiffness in the joints, which can make everyday movements like walking, writing, or gripping objects more difficult. This is often worse in the morning or after periods of inactivity.

5. *Skin Dryness:* Dry, flaky skin that may be accompanied by rashes, itching, or irritation. This can sometimes lead to cracks in the skin, making it more susceptible to infections or discomfort.

6. *Fatigue:* Persistent, overwhelming tiredness that doesn't improve with rest. This fatigue can impact daily activities, making it hard to concentrate, maintain energy, or stay productive throughout the day.

Other symptoms can include dry throat, dry cough, and vaginal dryness. It's important to consult a healthcare professional for a proper diagnosis and treatment plan if you suspect you have Sjogren's Syndrome.

Each individual's experience with Sjogren's varies, and symptom severity can differ from mild irritation to major complications like corneal damage or even non-Hodgkin's lymphoma, a rare but serious development in some cases.

Causes

The exact cause of Sjogren's Syndrome is unknown, but it is an autoimmune disease where the immune system attacks healthy tissues. Researchers believe it stems from a mix of genetic, environmental factors, and immune dysfunction.

- *Autoimmune Mechanism:* Sjogren's Syndrome occurs when the immune system attacks exocrine glands, reducing saliva and tear production. It can also affect other organs like joints, lungs, kidneys, liver, or skin, causing additional symptoms and complications.
- *Genetic Influences:* Research shows a genetic link to Sjogren's Syndrome. Certain immune system genes may increase risk, and it often runs in families with autoimmune diseases like lupus or rheumatoid arthritis.
- *Environmental Triggers:* Genes play a role, but environmental factors often trigger Sjogren's Syndrome in susceptible individuals. Viruses, infections, stress, or toxic chemicals can activate the

immune system and cause dysfunction. Researchers are still studying which factors matter most.

With a better understanding of the causes, doctors can develop more targeted treatments. But for now, Sjogren's Syndrome remains an enigma with no clear cure.

Risk Factors

Certain risk factors are known to increase the likelihood of developing the disease.

1. *Age:* Sjogren's Syndrome is most commonly diagnosed in individuals over the age of 40, although it can occur at any age. This autoimmune condition tends to develop later in life, often affecting middle-aged and older adults, with women being more frequently diagnosed than men.

2. *Gender:* Women are disproportionately affected, making up 90% of diagnoses. Hormonal differences and fluctuations may play a role in this disparity.

3. *Family History:* Having a close family member with an autoimmune disorder can increase the risk of developing Sjogren's Syndrome or another autoimmune disease.

4. *Coexisting Autoimmune Disorders:* Many people with Sjogren's also have another autoimmune disease, such as rheumatoid arthritis or lupus. This overlap often complicates diagnosis and management.

Understanding the origins and mechanisms of Sjogren's Syndrome is vital, not just for those diagnosed but for their families, caregivers, and the healthcare community. While there's currently no cure, ongoing research and improved therapies provide hope for better symptom management and a higher standard of living.

Diagnosing Sjogren's Syndrome

Diagnosing Sjogren's Syndrome can be challenging because no single test can confirm its presence. Instead, healthcare providers rely on a combination of symptom evaluation, medical history, physical examination, and laboratory tests to arrive at a diagnosis. This comprehensive approach helps identify the condition while ruling out other potential causes of symptoms.

Symptoms

The diagnostic process often begins with identifying the symptoms most commonly associated with Sjogren's Syndrome. These include:

- *Dryness of the Eyes:* A gritty, burning sensation, redness, blurred vision, and light sensitivity are frequent complaints.
- *Dryness of the Mouth:* A sticky feeling in the mouth, difficulty swallowing, cracked lips, and frequent thirst are common. A dry mouth raises the risk of cavities, gum disease, and oral infections.

- *Systemic Symptoms:* Joint pain, skin rashes, severe fatigue, and swelling of the salivary glands may also appear.

Recognizing these symptoms is key to initiating the diagnostic process.

Medical History

A detailed medical history forms the foundation of diagnosis. Your doctor will ask about the nature and duration of your symptoms, such as the severity of dryness or fatigue. They'll also gather information about:

- *Family History:* Any relatives with Sjogren's Syndrome or other autoimmune conditions.
- *Personal Medical History:* Previous diagnoses of autoimmune diseases or related conditions, such as rheumatoid arthritis or lupus.

Environmental or Lifestyle Factors: Any factors that might trigger or worsen your symptoms, such as specific medications or previous infections.

This step helps guide further tests by identifying potential patterns or risks specific to Sjogren's Syndrome.

Physical Examination

During a physical exam, the doctor will look for telltale signs of Sjogren's Syndrome. This might include:

- ***Mouth Examination:*** Checking for dryness (such as stickiness or cracked lips), signs of oral infections, or swollen salivary glands. They may also ask about difficulties chewing or swallowing.
- ***Eye Examination:*** Observing the eyes for redness, irritation, or tear deficiency. Patients might report a gritty or burning sensation.
- ***General Symptoms:*** Swollen joints, skin rashes, or extreme fatigue indicative of systemic involvement.

Based on findings from the physical exam, additional diagnostic tests may be ordered to confirm the condition.

Laboratory and Diagnostic Tests

To gain a clearer picture, medical professionals use several specialized tests. Each test plays a vital role in assessing gland function, immune markers, and inflammation levels:

1. **Salivary Gland Function Tests**
   - ***Sialometry:*** Measures the flow rate of saliva. Reduced production is a strong indicator of salivary gland dysfunction.
   - ***Sialography:*** Uses X-rays to visualize the salivary glands and detect blockages, inflammation, or structural abnormalities.
2. **Tear Function Tests**
   - ***Schirmer's Test:*** A small strip of paper is placed under the eyelid to measure tear

production. Reduced tear output can indicate gland dysfunction.

- *Tear Film Break-up Time:* Assesses how long the tear film remains stable before it breaks, suggesting dryness severity.

3. Blood Tests

Blood tests can detect a range of markers associated with autoimmune diseases, including:

- *Anti-SSA (Ro) and Anti-SSB (La):* Autoantibodies closely linked to Sjogren's Syndrome and commonly used in diagnosis.
- *Rheumatoid Factor (RF):* Often present in people with Sjogren's Syndrome, even without rheumatoid arthritis.
- *Elevated Erythrocyte Sedimentation Rate (ESR) or C-Reactive Protein (CRP):* Indicates inflammation.
- *Lip Biopsy:* A small sample of tissue is taken from inside the lip and examined under a microscope. This test looks for glandular inflammation and damage, which are hallmark features of Sjogren's Syndrome. Lip biopsy is particularly helpful when other test results are inconclusive.
- *Imaging Tests:* Imaging studies may be used to evaluate gland structure and function:

- *Ultrasound or MRI:* Provides detailed images of the salivary glands, helping to identify inflammation, enlargement, or cysts.
- *CT Scans:* Offer a broader view to assess damage or inflammation in connected tissues or organs.

Diagnosing Sjogren's Syndrome involves evaluating symptoms, physical exams, and lab tests to ensure accuracy and prevent misdiagnosis. Early diagnosis is crucial to avoid complications like infections or organ damage and improve quality of life through timely treatment. A comprehensive approach helps healthcare providers deliver personalized and effective care.

Women and Sjogren's Syndrome

Sjogren's Syndrome disproportionately affects women, with females being up to ten times more likely to develop the condition than men. Although the disease can occur at any age, it is most commonly diagnosed in women over 40. This striking gender disparity has intrigued researchers and led to exploration into the underlying reasons why women are more susceptible to Sjogren's Syndrome.

Why Women Are More Affected

There is no single explanation for why women experience Sjogren's Syndrome at significantly higher rates than men. However, several theories attempt to shed light on this gender difference:

1. **Hormonal Factors**

   The female hormone estrogen is thought to play a central role. Estrogen levels fluctuate throughout a woman's life—during the menstrual cycle, pregnancy, and menopause. These fluctuations may influence the immune system, making it more prone to autoimmunity.

Interestingly, women with Sjogren's Syndrome often report a worsening of symptoms during periods of high estrogen, such as during certain phases of their menstrual cycle. Additionally, the decline of estrogen during menopause is believed to contribute to the onset or progression of the disease, further supporting the hormone's connection to Sjogren's.

2. Immune System Variations

Women tend to have a more responsive immune system compared to men, which helps them fight infections more efficiently. However, this heightened immune activity may also make their immune systems more likely to mistake the body's own tissues as invaders, leading to autoimmune diseases like Sjogren's Syndrome.

3. Genetic and Environmental Factors

Genetics may predispose women to autoimmune conditions, and certain genes influencing the immune response could be more active in females. Additionally, environmental triggers—such as viral infections—may initiate autoimmune responses differently in women due to their hormonal or genetic makeup.

Regardless of the specific cause, Sjogren's Syndrome remains a significant health concern for women. While this chronic condition can be challenging, proper treatment and management allow most women to lead fulfilling, relatively normal lives.

Treatment Options for Sjogren's Syndrome

Although there is no cure for Sjogren's Syndrome, various treatments focus on relieving symptoms, preventing complications, and improving quality of life. Treatment plans often combine medications, lifestyle changes, and, in rare cases, surgical interventions to address the diverse symptoms of the disease.

1. **Artificial Tears and Saliva**

   Dry eyes and dry mouth are hallmark symptoms of Sjogren's Syndrome, and using artificial tears or saliva substitutes can bring significant relief.

   - *Artificial Tears:* These eyedrops lubricate the eyes, reduce irritation, and help prevent secondary issues like eye infections or corneal damage.
   - *Saliva Substitutes:* Over-the-counter sprays, gels, or lozenges can moisten the mouth, ease discomfort, and reduce the risk of gum disease or cavities.

Both treatments are easy to use and provide essential symptom relief, making daily life more manageable.

2. Anti-Inflammatory Medications

Nonsteroidal anti-inflammatory drugs (NSAIDs) like ibuprofen are often used to control inflammation, particularly in the joints. They can also help combat headaches and general discomfort associated with the condition.

- *Pros:* NSAIDs are widely available and effective for mild to moderate symptoms.
- *Cons:* Prolonged use can lead to side effects like stomach upset, gastrointestinal bleeding, or kidney problems. Always consult a doctor before taking NSAIDs regularly.

3. Immunosuppressive Medications

For more severe cases, immunosuppressive drugs may be prescribed. These medications dampen the immune system's activity, reducing inflammation and limiting damage to the glands and other tissues.

- Examples include hydroxychloroquine, often used for systemic symptoms or more potent options like methotrexate or biologic agents.
- While these drugs can significantly improve quality of life, they come with potential side effects, such as increased vulnerability to

infections. Therefore, they require close monitoring by a healthcare provider.

4. Surgery

Though uncommon, surgical interventions may be necessary for severe complications.

- Salivary Gland Surgery: Damage to the salivary glands could require corrective procedures.
- Punctal Occlusion: A minor surgery to block tear ducts, which helps retain natural tears and reduce eye dryness.

Surgery is typically reserved for cases where other treatments have not provided relief.

5. Lifestyle Changes

Implementing small lifestyle adjustments can have a big impact on managing symptoms and improving overall well-being.

- *Hydration:* Drinking plenty of water throughout the day can maintain moisture levels in the mouth and throat.
- *Humidifiers:* Adding moisture to the air can alleviate dry eyes, skin, and nasal passages, especially in arid or air-conditioned environments.

- *Avoiding Irritants:* Reducing exposure to smoke, wind, and other environmental factors can prevent symptoms from worsening.

Other tactics, like getting enough rest, eating a balanced diet, and avoiding overly dry foods or drinks, can also improve symptom management and quality of life.

Sjogren's Syndrome affects women more often due to hormonal, genetic, and immune factors, causing symptoms like dryness, joint pain, and fatigue. While there's no cure, early diagnosis, personalized treatments, and proper support can help manage symptoms, prevent complications, and enable women to lead active, fulfilling lives.

Challenges in Childbearing and Parenting with Sjogren's Syndrome

Parenting with Sjogren's Syndrome presents unique challenges, from pregnancy and breastfeeding to managing fatigue. This chapter offers strategies and insights to help individuals navigate these hurdles and make informed decisions throughout their parenting journey.

Insights into Pregnancy and Breastfeeding Challenges

The decision to have children while managing Sjogren's Syndrome often raises many questions about health, medications, and energy levels. Here are some key factors to consider:

Pregnancy and Sjogren's Syndrome

- *Pregnancy Risks:* Pregnancy with Sjogren's is often successful but may carry risks like miscarriage, preterm birth, or low birth weight. Antibodies such as

SSA/Ro and SSB/La can increase the chance of neonatal lupus or congenital heart block in newborns.

- *Specialized Care:* Working closely with a rheumatologist, obstetrician, and potentially a maternal-fetal medicine specialist is essential for monitoring both your health and your baby's. Frequent checkups throughout the pregnancy ensure that any complications are detected early.

Breastfeeding with Sjogren's

- *Impact of Dryness:* One challenge unique to individuals with Sjogren's is the potential for insufficient milk production due to glandular dysfunction. Keep in mind that supplementing with formula, if needed, does not diminish the meaningful bond created during feeding.
- *Medication Considerations:* Some medications used to treat Sjogren's may not be safe while breastfeeding. Discussing alternative treatments with your healthcare provider can help ensure both you and your baby's safety during this period.

Potential Impact of Sjogren's Medications on Pregnancy and Breastfeeding

Medications play a key role in managing Sjogren's symptoms, but not all are safe during pregnancy or breastfeeding. It's crucial to collaborate with your healthcare team to tailor a treatment plan before conceiving:

- **Safe Medications:** Hydroxychloroquine (Plaquenil) is often considered safe during pregnancy and can help manage fatigue, joint pain, and inflammation.
- **Avoided Medications:** Certain drugs, such as methotrexate and mycophenolate mofetil, should be discontinued before conception due to risks of miscarriage and birth defects.
- **Tapering off Immunosuppressants:** If immunosuppressants are part of your treatment, your doctor may recommend transitioning to milder alternatives or closely monitoring your dosage to minimize risks.
- **Breastfeeding Safety:** Medications such as corticosteroids may require careful timing to avoid peak concentrations in breast milk. Working with a lactation consultant can help balance managing your symptoms with breastfeeding goals.

Balancing Energy Levels and Managing Fatigue While Parenting

Parenting demands energy and attention, which may feel particularly challenging when grappling with the chronic fatigue associated with Sjogren's. While there's no one-size-fits-all solution, these strategies can help:

1. ***Build a Daily Routine:*** Plan parenting tasks around your peak energy times and include rest breaks during the day to recharge.
2. ***Simplify Tasks:*** Share household tasks with others and use services like meal kits or grocery delivery to simplify daily responsibilities.
3. ***Practice Gentle Parenting Techniques:*** Try low-energy parenting activities like reading, puzzles, crafts, or educational shows to bond with your child while conserving energy.
4. ***Promote Physical Health:*** Maintain a healthy lifestyle with anti-inflammatory foods, hydration, and moderate exercise like yoga or stretching to boost energy and well-being.
5. ***Share the Load:*** Rely on your support system, including co-parents, grandparents, or trusted caregivers, to help share responsibilities.

Tips for Parenting Decisions Based on Health Awareness

Parenting with a chronic condition like Sjogren's requires thoughtful planning and self-awareness to maintain both your health and your child's needs.

1. Be Honest About Limitations

Open up to your children about your energy levels in a way they can understand. For example, saying,

"Mommy needs a rest for a little while so she can play with you later," helps them develop empathy without feeling neglected.

2. Prioritize Quality Time Over Quantity

Focus on meaningful activities that align with your energy. A few minutes of engaged play or conversation can have a lasting impact.

3. Make Advance Plans for Flares

Create backup plans for days when fatigue or symptoms are more intense. Keep a list of low-energy activities like books, podcasts, or creative play that older children can enjoy independently, and have ready-to-eat meals stocked.

4. Teach Independence Early

Encourage your children to take small, age-appropriate responsibilities. Tasks like tidying up their toys or helping with minor household tasks can foster independence while alleviating some of your daily workload.

5. Build a Village

Establish a network of reliable caregivers who can provide extra support, whether it's a trusted neighbor, family member, or a part-time nanny.

Parenting with Sjogren's Syndrome can be tough, but with support, self-care, and open communication with your healthcare team, it's manageable. Prioritize meaningful connections and accept help to create a positive experience.

The Connection Between Sjogren's Syndrome and Other Autoimmune Diseases

Sjogren's Syndrome often overlaps with other autoimmune diseases like lupus and rheumatoid arthritis, making diagnosis and management more complex. Understanding these connections is key to improving health and quality of life.

Common Autoimmune Diseases Linked to Sjogren's Syndrome

Research shows that people with Sjogren's Syndrome are more likely to develop other autoimmune conditions. Some of the most commonly associated diseases include the following:

- *Lupus (Systemic Lupus Erythematosus):* Lupus is a systemic autoimmune disorder that, like Sjogren's, causes joint pain, fatigue, and inflammation. Both conditions are more common in women and result from the immune system attacking the body's own tissues.

- **Rheumatoid Arthritis (RA):** RA causes joint inflammation, swelling, and pain, often leading to secondary Sjogren's Syndrome, which impacts glands responsible for producing moisture, intensifying symptoms.
- **Hashimoto's Thyroiditis:** This autoimmune condition affects the thyroid, causing hypothyroidism with symptoms like fatigue, dry skin, and hair loss, which can resemble those of Sjogren's Syndrome.
- **Scleroderma:** Scleroderma results in the hardening and thickening of the skin and connective tissue. When paired with Sjogren's, it can exacerbate dryness and joint stiffness.
- **Primary Biliary Cholangitis (PBC):** PBC affects the liver, causing bile duct inflammation. Like Sjogren's, it is an organ-specific autoimmune disorder that may present with symptoms such as dry eyes and fatigue.

The coexistence of these conditions emphasizes the systemic nature of autoimmune diseases and highlights the importance of looking beyond isolated symptoms.

How Overlapping Symptoms Complicate Diagnosis

Many autoimmune diseases share similar symptoms, such as fatigue, joint pain, and dryness. This overlap can make pinpointing a diagnosis difficult, often leading to delays in treatment. For instance:

- *Fatigue and Joint Pain:* Both lupus and rheumatoid arthritis often cause fatigue and inflammation similar to Sjogren's, leading to misdiagnosis or underdiagnosis.
- *Dryness Symptoms:* Dry eyes and dry mouth, hallmark symptoms of Sjogren's, may also be present in lupus or mixed connective tissue disorders.
- *Organ-Specific Complications:* Kidney involvement in lupus or liver issues in primary biliary cholangitis can distract from a diagnosis of Sjogren's, even when dryness symptoms are present.

Diagnosing Sjogren's often involves a team of specialists and tests like autoantibody blood work and salivary gland biopsies to differentiate it from similar conditions.

Mental Health and Emotional Coping with Sjogren's Syndrome

Living with Sjogren's Syndrome affects both physical and mental health. Its chronic and unpredictable nature can impact emotional well-being, but focusing on mental health can help manage symptoms more effectively.

The Psychological Impact of Chronic Illness

Adjusting to life with Sjogren's Syndrome often means navigating feelings of anxiety, depression, and even social isolation. These mental health challenges are common among those with chronic conditions due to their impact on daily life.

- *Anxiety:* Uncertainty over disease progression, treatment outcomes, or day-to-day discomfort can lead to heightened feelings of worry or even panic.
- *Depression:* Persistent fatigue, dryness, and pain, combined with the feeling that Sjogren's limits one's life, can trigger depression. Symptoms may include a constant sense of sadness, reduced energy, or loss of interest in previously enjoyable activities.

- *Social Isolation:* Chronic illnesses often make socializing more difficult, whether due to physical limitations, exhaustion, or the fear of feeling burdened by others. Over time, this can lead to feelings of loneliness or disconnection.

Acknowledging these challenges is the first step toward addressing them and improving overall mental health.

Practical Coping Strategies

Coping with the emotional toll of Sjogren's starts with taking proactive steps to care for your mental well-being. While each person's experience is unique, the following strategies can contribute to a more balanced emotional state.

1. **Therapy and Counseling**

   Talking to a licensed therapist or counselor can be immensely beneficial.

   - *Cognitive Behavioral Therapy (CBT):* This is a structured form of therapy that helps people identify and change negative thought patterns that contribute to anxiety or depression.
   - *Acceptance and Commitment Therapy (ACT):* ACT focuses on accepting life's challenges while committing to actions that align with your present values—this can be particularly

empowering for those living with chronic illness.

- *Grief Counseling:* Adjusting to a new reality with Sjogren can lead to a sense of loss. Counseling can help process these emotions and build resilience.

2. **Mindfulness Practices and Stress Management**

Stress can worsen autoimmune symptoms by increasing inflammation and fatigue while reducing emotional resilience. Mindfulness practices help manage stress and restore calm.

- *Meditation:* Regular mindfulness or guided meditation can help reduce anxiety and bring attention back to the present moment. Apps like Calm or Headspace often have chronic illness-specific meditations.
- *Breathing Exercises:* Simple techniques, such as abdominal breathing or the 4-7-8 method (inhaling for 4 seconds, holding for 7, exhaling for 8), can lower stress levels in minutes.
- *Yoga or Gentle Movement:* Slow, intentional movement paired with mindful breathing not only helps manage stress but can also relieve stiffness and tension in the body.

3. Stay Active Within Your Limits

Physical activity releases endorphins, the body's natural mood boosters. Even with limited energy, small acts of movement can make a big difference—like gentle stretching, short walks, or tai chi. These activities also promote better sleep and combat the lethargy that can accompany depression.

4. Engage in Creative Outlets

Expressive activities like journaling, painting, or gardening can help process emotions and bring a sense of accomplishment. Keeping a gratitude journal, in particular, has been shown to improve mood by focusing attention on positive aspects of your day, however small they may seem.

5. Plan for Social Connection

Staying socially connected, even in small ways, can reduce feelings of isolation. Make time for virtual chats, short meet-ups with friends, or even online interactions within communities where others understand your challenges.

Self-care is essential for managing chronic illness. Be compassionate and flexible, adapting to your body's needs. Seeking support from a therapist or group can help, reminding you that you're not alone and better days are possible.

Supporting Families and Caregivers

Caring for someone with Sjogren's Syndrome can be challenging but rewarding. This condition, with symptoms like fatigue, dryness, and joint pain, impacts both the individual and their caregivers. Understanding the condition and adopting effective strategies can help create a supportive environment for everyone involved.

Tips for Providing Emotional and Practical Support

Supporting someone with a chronic illness like Sjogren's requires both emotional understanding and practical assistance. Here are some simple but impactful ways to offer your care:

1. **Be a Compassionate Listener**
   - Allow your loved one to express their feelings without judgment. Listen actively and validate their experiences. For example, instead of

offering solutions immediately, say, "That sounds really difficult. I'm here for you."

- Acknowledge their feelings of frustration, sadness, or fatigue—sometimes, just being heard can make a world of difference.

2. **Offer Practical Assistance**

- Help with daily tasks that may feel overwhelming. Simple gestures like preparing meals, assisting with grocery shopping, or accompanying them to doctor's appointments can ease their burden.
- Encourage them to conserve their energy for activities they enjoy by taking on tasks they find exhausting.

3. **Encourage Self-Care**

- Gently remind your loved one to hydrate, use moisturizing eye drops, and follow any other treatments prescribed by their healthcare provider.
- Support them in prioritizing rest, which is vital, especially on days when fatigue is more pronounced.

4. **Respect Their Individual Needs**

- Recognize that symptoms may vary day-to-day. Avoid making assumptions about what they can or can't do. Instead, ask, "What would be most helpful for you today?"

- Allow them the space and time to communicate their needs.

Being emotionally and practically supportive means understanding that your loved one's experience with Sjogren is unique and may change day to day. Your willingness to listen, assist, and encourage self-care can help them manage their illness more effectively.

Strategies for Open Communication and Establishing Boundaries

Effective communication fosters a healthy dynamic between you and your loved one while also setting necessary boundaries to maintain everyone's well-being.

1. **Keep Communication Open and Honest**
   - Regularly check in with your loved one about how they're feeling—both physically and emotionally. This creates an open channel for dialogue.
   - Share your own experiences and feelings where appropriate, so they don't feel like they are the only ones struggling.
   - If you're uncertain about how to help, don't hesitate to ask. Questions like, "What can I do to make things easier?" show that you care and are willing to learn.

2. Respect Personal Boundaries

- Understand that managing a chronic illness can be overwhelming. Respect your loved one's need for privacy or alone time if they express it.
- Likewise, set boundaries for yourself to avoid burnout. Communicate your own limits kindly. For instance, say, "I want to help you the best I can, but I need to take some time for myself in the evenings to recharge."

3. Be Patient in Difficult Conversations

- Chronic illnesses can affect mood and emotions. Approach conversations with patience, even if your loved one is feeling irritable or withdrawn.
- Avoid blaming language or frustration, as it may amplify their stress. Instead, shift to understanding comments, like, "I know today's been tough, and I'm here if you need a break."

By practicing open communication and setting boundaries, you can support your loved one while also taking care of yourself. Remember to be patient, understanding, and most importantly, always listen to their needs.

Empathy, Patience, and Self-Care for Caregivers

Caring for someone with a chronic illness is a selfless role, but it can also be emotionally and physically draining. Prioritizing your own well-being equips you to provide better care in the long run.

1. **Practice Empathy and Patience**
   - Put yourself in their shoes—imagine the challenges they face daily, and use that perspective to deepen your empathy.
   - Cultivate patience. Chronic conditions come with ups and downs, so understanding that their needs will change over time is key.

2. **Don't Neglect Your Own Needs**
   - Take regular breaks from caregiving to focus on activities that rejuvenate you, such as hobbies, exercise, or spending time with friends.
   - Seek respite care or ask other family members to alternate caregiving duties, so you don't carry the full responsibility alone.
   - Watch for signs of caregiver burnout, such as fatigue, irritability, or feeling overwhelmed, and address these feelings proactively.

3. **Join Caregiver Support Groups**
   - Engaging with other caregivers who understand your challenges can provide emotional relief.

They may also share tips and resources that can help you better manage your role.

- Online forums or in-person groups offer convenient ways to exchange ideas and build a sense of community.
- Supporting someone with Sjogren's Syndrome involves empathy, open communication, and self-care. Understanding their condition and fostering dialogue can improve their well-being while prioritizing your own health helps you remain a strong source of support.

Managing Sjogren's Syndrome Through Diet

While there is no cure for Sjogren's Syndrome, diet can play a key role in managing its symptoms and improving overall quality of life. The foods you eat (or avoid) can impact inflammation levels, energy, and the severity of dryness. This guide outlines dietary adjustments that can help ease symptoms while supporting overall health.

The Role of Diet in Symptom Management

Sjogren's Syndrome often causes widespread inflammation and dryness, which can lead to fatigue, mouth sores, and joint pain. A well-balanced diet rich in anti-inflammatory and antioxidant foods can help address these issues. At the same time, avoiding inflammatory or irritative foods can reduce symptom flare-ups and discomfort.

Foods to Eat

Focusing on nutrient-dense, anti-inflammatory, and hydrating foods is essential for those managing Sjogren's Syndrome. These foods can help reduce inflammation, support immune function, and maintain hydration for the tissues affected by dryness.

1. *Antioxidant-Rich Foods*

Antioxidants combat free radicals, which can damage cells and contribute to inflammation. Including more antioxidants in your diet can help protect against tissue damage and alleviate symptoms.

- Leafy Greens: Kale, Swiss chard, and spinach.
- Berries: Strawberries, blueberries, and raspberries are packed with potent antioxidants.
- Nuts and Seeds: Almonds, walnuts, and flaxseeds.
- Whole Grains: Brown rice, quinoa, and oats are rich in valuable phytonutrients.

While antioxidants can also be taken in supplement form, getting them from whole foods ensures you benefit from other vitamins and minerals naturally present in these foods.

2. *Anti-Inflammatory Foods*

Chronic inflammation worsens many symptoms of Sjogren's Syndrome, especially joint pain and fatigue. Foods with anti-inflammatory properties can help calm this response.

- Turmeric and Ginger: Both contain potent anti-inflammatory compounds.
- Garlic: Promotes immune health while reducing inflammation.
- Fatty Fish: Salmon, mackerel, and tuna are high in omega-3s, and known for their inflammation-fighting properties.
- Olive Oil: A healthy fat that benefits heart health and reduces inflammatory markers.
- Nuts and Seeds: Almonds, walnuts, and chia seeds not only provide anti-inflammatory benefits but also support moisture retention.
- Green Tea: Contains antioxidants and compounds that reduce inflammation.

Adding these foods regularly as part of meals or snacks can make a noticeable difference in symptom management.

3. *Staying Hydrated*

Hydration is crucial for managing dryness associated with Sjogren's Syndrome. While water is the best option, incorporating water-rich foods like cucumbers, watermelon, and celery can supplement hydration.

Foods to Avoid

Certain foods can exacerbate symptoms or contribute to inflammation, making it important to minimize or avoid these triggers.

1. ***Sugary Foods and Drinks:*** Sugar is a major contributor to inflammation and can worsen symptoms like dryness and oral discomfort.
   - Avoid candies, cookies, cakes, and other sugary treats.
   - Limit sugary beverages such as sodas, energy drinks, and fruit juices.

   Reducing sugar intake not only mitigates symptoms but also protects against dental decay and gum disease, which people with Sjogren's Syndrome are more susceptible to.

2. ***Saturated Fats:*** Foods high in saturated fats, like fatty red meats, butter, and full-fat dairy, can potentially lead to inflammation and weight gain, adding extra strain to the joints.

3. ***Refined Carbohydrates:*** Processed carbs, such as white bread, pastries, and chips, can cause blood sugar spikes and promote systemic inflammation. Opt for whole grains to keep energy levels stable.

4. ***Alcohol:*** Alcohol exacerbates dryness, including in the mouth and throat, and can interfere with the body's

moisture absorption. Limiting or avoiding alcohol can help manage these symptoms.

5. *Caffeinated Beverages:* Caffeine acts as a diuretic, potentially leading to dehydration. While small amounts may be fine for some people, excessive caffeine in coffee, tea, and energy drinks can worsen symptoms of dryness.

6. *Spicy Foods:* Foods with strong spices often trigger saliva and tear production, which can paradoxically lead to more dryness and even irritate the gastrointestinal tract.

7. *Acidic Foods:* Tomatoes, citrus fruits, and vinegar-based products can irritate the mucous membranes and lead to mouth sores, making it difficult to eat or swallow.

Planning a Balanced Diet

When managing Sjogren's Syndrome, striking the right balance between anti-inflammatory and antioxidant foods while eliminating potential irritants is key. A typical day might include meals such as:

- *Breakfast:* Whole-grain oatmeal topped with fresh berries and a handful of nuts.
- *Lunch:* A spinach and kale salad with grilled salmon, olive oil, and turmeric dressing.

- *Snack:* Green tea and a small portion of almonds or walnuts.
- *Dinner:* Baked chicken or tofu, quinoa, and steamed vegetables like broccoli and carrots.

Before making significant changes to your diet, consult your healthcare provider or a registered dietitian. They can help tailor a plan to your unique needs, ensuring you get the right balance of nutrients without compromising on other aspects of health.

Dietary changes are not a cure for Sjogren's Syndrome, but they can be a powerful tool for managing symptoms and enhancing well-being. By focusing on nutrient-rich, anti-inflammatory foods and avoiding known irritants, you can support your body's efforts to fight inflammation, reduce dryness, and maintain energy levels. Combine these changes with medical treatments and other self-care strategies to achieve the best possible quality of life.

3-Step Plan for Implementing This Diet

If you're ready to start managing your Sjogren's syndrome through diet, here's a 3-step plan for getting started:

Step 1: Learn About the Sjogren's Syndrome Diet

The first step in leveraging diet to help manage Sjogren's Syndrome symptoms is to educate yourself about the foods that can either alleviate or exacerbate your condition. This foundational knowledge empowers you to make informed choices, adopt healthier eating habits, and ultimately improve your quality of life.

Understand the Role of Diet in Symptom Management

Sjogren's Syndrome affects various systems in the body, including the immune and exocrine systems, which are responsible for producing moisture (such as saliva and tears). Certain foods can reduce inflammation, protect cells from damage, and support hydration, while others may trigger flare-ups or worsen dryness and fatigue.

Knowing how your diet interacts with your symptoms is essential. It's not just about eating well—it's about eating with purpose to minimize discomfort and optimize your body's health.

How to Research Effectively

When learning about the Sjogren's Syndrome diet, it's important to rely on accurate and trustworthy information. Here are some steps to guide your research process:

1. *Look for Reliable Online Sources:*

Start with reputable websites that provide evidence-based information on autoimmune diseases. Resources affiliated with medical organizations, research institutions, or government health agencies—such as the National Institutes of Health (NIH) or the American College of Rheumatology—are excellent places to begin. Avoid blogs or forums that lack scientific backing, as misinformation could lead to improper dietary choices.

2. *Explore Scientific Studies:*

Look for peer-reviewed journal articles or clinical research focused on autoimmune diseases and dietary interventions. These studies can shed light on how certain foods influence inflammation markers or hydration levels in the body.

3. Seek Community Support:

Join support groups or communities for individuals with Sjogren's Syndrome. Online forums and local meetups can provide firsthand experiences about what dietary changes work for others. While these anecdotes should not replace medical advice, they can offer practical insights or food ideas to explore.

4. Check Ingredients and Labels:

Educate yourself on how to read nutritional labels and identify ingredients that may either benefit or trigger symptoms. For example, excessive sugar, refined carbohydrates, or trans fats might worsen inflammation, while omega-3 fatty acids and antioxidants can support symptom relief.

Consulting Healthcare Professionals

While learning independently is valuable, consulting experts ensure you're receiving tailored, accurate advice:

1. Talk to Your Doctor:

Your doctor is the first point of contact for any questions about managing symptoms through diet. They can discuss the specific dietary needs of people with Sjogren's Syndrome and may perform tests to identify deficiencies or sensitivities.

2. **Partner with a Registered Dietitian:**

   A registered dietitian specializes in nutrition and can assess your specific needs and preferences. They will help create a personalized dietary plan that considers your unique symptoms, medical history, and lifestyle. For instance, if dry mouth makes swallowing difficult, they can suggest soft or hydrating foods that are easier to consume without exacerbating irritation.

3. **Specialists and Multidisciplinary Care: If needed, a rheumatologist or immunologist can provide additional guidance on how diet interacts with medications or treatments you're undergoing for Sjogren's Syndrome.**

Benefits of Personalized Dietary Plans

The "one-size-fits-all" approach does not apply to managing Sjogren's Syndrome through diet. Personalizing your diet ensures that you target your specific symptoms while also meeting your body's nutritional needs. For example:

- If joint pain is a key issue, your dietitian might emphasize anti-inflammatory foods such as salmon, turmeric, or olive oil.
- If energy is a concern, they might suggest reducing simple carbohydrates and incorporating slow-digesting whole grains and healthy fats to maintain stable blood sugar levels.

- Those with significant dryness might benefit from including water-rich foods like cucumbers and melons or identifying safe beverages that aid hydration without contributing to dryness.

Educating yourself about the dietary aspects of Sjogren's Syndrome can boost your confidence and help you manage symptoms alongside medical treatments. Understanding the link between diet and autoimmune health encourages healthier eating habits and better communication with healthcare providers.

By learning the basics, you can start incorporating Sjogren's-friendly foods into your routine, staying patient as benefits take time. With the right knowledge and commitment, your diet can become a powerful tool for managing symptoms and improving your quality of life.

Step 2: Incorporate More of the Recommended Foods Into Your Diet

Now that you've learned which foods can help manage Sjogren's Syndrome symptoms, the next step is integrating them into your daily routine. Making dietary changes doesn't have to be overwhelming or drastic. By starting small and building on those changes, you can seamlessly adopt a healthier diet that supports your well-being over time.

1. **Start Small with Simple Changes**

   Making gradual adjustments to your diet ensures that the changes are sustainable. Here are some practical ways to start incorporating anti-inflammatory and antioxidant-rich foods into your meals without feeling overburdened:

   - *Add More Vegetables to Your Plates:* Start by including an extra serving of leafy greens or colorful vegetables at each meal. For example, pair your sandwich with a spinach side salad or add sautéed broccoli to your pasta dishes.
   - *Swap Snacks for Nutrient-Dense Options:* Replace processed snack foods like chips with a handful of almonds, walnuts, or fresh berries for a more nourishing alternative.
   - *Enhance Breakfast with Superfoods:* Stir some flaxseed, chia seeds, or fresh fruit into your morning oatmeal or yogurt to boost antioxidants and omega-3s.
   - *Use Spices in Your Cooking:* Add turmeric, ginger, or garlic to soups, stir-fries, or roasted veggies. These spices are packed with anti-inflammatory properties and instantly elevate the taste of your meals.

These smaller changes allow you to experiment with flavors and find what works best for your tastes and symptoms.

2. Plan Your Meals to Stay on Track

Meal planning is an effective way to ensure you're consistently incorporating the recommended foods into your diet. Preparation helps you avoid relying on unhealthy, inflammatory options when you're short on time.

- *Create a Weekly Menu:* Plan meals that include anti-inflammatory ingredients like salmon, kale, and olive oil. For instance, a menu might feature grilled salmon with quinoa and roasted sweet potatoes for dinner or a spinach and berry smoothie for breakfast.
- *Batch Cook for Convenience:* Cook larger portions of healthy meals like stews, soups, or roasted vegetables, and refrigerate or freeze portions for the week.
- *Balance Your Plate:* Use the half-plate method—fill half your plate with vegetables, a quarter with a lean protein like fatty fish or chicken, and the final quarter with whole grains like brown rice or quinoa.

Keeping your meals varied and flavorful prevents boredom and makes it easier to stick with your new eating habits.

3. Shop Smart for Success

Stocking your kitchen with the right ingredients is key to healthier eating habits. Here are some tips for grocery shopping with Sjogren's Syndrome in mind:

- *Make a Shopping List:* Start with a list of anti-inflammatory and antioxidant-rich foods, such as berries, leafy greens, nuts, seeds, fatty fish, and olive oil. Avoid buying processed or sugary snacks by sticking to your list.
- *Shop the Perimeter:* The outer aisles of grocery stores usually contain fresh produce, lean proteins, and whole foods, while the inner aisles often house processed and packaged items. Focus your time on the produce and fresh meat or fish sections.
- *Read Labels Carefully:* When purchasing packaged products like salad dressings or snacks, check for added sugars, unhealthy fats, or artificial ingredients. Choose simple, whole-food options whenever possible.
- *Buy in Bulk:* Nuts, seeds, and grains can often be purchased in bulk at lower prices. Keep a

supply of these staples at home to add to salads, breakfasts, or smoothies.

4. Experiment in the Kitchen

Cooking at home is one of the best ways to take control of your diet and manage symptoms. Here's how to make the transition smooth and enjoyable:

- *Try New Recipes:* Look for recipes that incorporate the foods recommended for Sjogren's Syndrome. For example, a vibrant turmeric-ginger carrot soup or a salmon and kale skillet dinner.
- *Use Swaps in Favorite Dishes:* Modify foods you already love. For example, replace white rice with quinoa or add avocado and olive oil instead of heavy dressings to salads.
- *Invest in Simple Tools:* A blender for smoothies, a spiralizer for vegetable noodles, or a slow cooker for batch cooking can make healthy eating more convenient.
- *Cook with Friends or Family:* Engaging loved ones in cooking can make the process less intimidating and more fun. Plus, sharing meals that meet your dietary goals sets a positive example for others.

5. Stay Consistent and Patient

Consistency is key when introducing new foods into your diet—but there's no need to rush the process. Adjusting to any dietary change takes time, and the benefits may not be immediate. Practice patience and focus on long-term progress by doing the following:

- *Set Realistic Goals:* Aim to try one or two new healthy foods each week instead of overhauling everything at once.
- *Track Your Progress:* Keep a food diary to note what you've eaten and how it made you feel. This can help you identify which foods work best for your symptoms.
- *Celebrate Small Wins:* Successfully swapping your morning pastry for a green smoothie or including more vegetables in your dinner is worth acknowledging. Every small step contributes to the bigger picture of improving your health.

6. Reevaluate and Refine Your Approach

Dietary needs can change over time, and not all foods work perfectly for everyone with Sjogren's Syndrome. Periodically reassess your progress and adjust your approach as needed:

- *Listen to Your Body:* Pay attention to how certain foods make you feel. If a recommended food doesn't sit well with you, discuss alternatives with your healthcare provider or dietitian.

- **Stay Flexible:** It's okay to adapt or modify your diet as you go. Dietary management is a personal and evolving process that may shift based on your symptoms or preferences.

Making dietary adjustments to manage Sjogren's Syndrome symptoms doesn't have to feel like an insurmountable challenge. By gradually introducing recommended foods, planning meals, and staying consistent, you can create a sustainable eating routine that truly supports your health.

With each small change, you're building toward a better quality of life, providing your body with the fuel it needs to fight inflammation and ease symptoms. Stay patient, enjoy the process, and celebrate the positive impact of nourishing your body.

Step 3: Avoid or Eliminate Problematic Foods From Your Diet

The final step in adapting your diet to manage Sjogren's Syndrome involves removing or reducing problematic foods that could trigger or worsen symptoms. Even with the best intentions, certain foods can contribute to inflammation, dehydrate the body, or aggravate dryness, fatigue, and joint pain. By addressing these triggers, you can take control of your symptoms and feel more comfortable in your daily life.

Identify Your Trigger Foods

The first step in avoiding problematic foods is identifying which ones impact your symptoms most. Since each person's experience with Sjogren's Syndrome is unique, not all trigger foods will affect you in the same way they affect others.

- *Observe Common Triggers:* Some of the most common culprits for symptom flare-ups include sugary foods, processed and refined carbs, high-saturated-fat foods, alcohol, caffeine, spicy dishes, and acidic foods. Take note if consuming these items coincides with worsened symptoms.
- *Track Your Diet:* Use a food diary to record what you eat and any symptoms you experience afterward. This can help you identify patterns and link specific foods to symptoms like increased dryness, joint pain, or fatigue.
- *Work With a Professional:* A registered dietitian or healthcare provider can guide you through elimination diets, where you systematically remove and reintroduce foods to pinpoint triggers.

Strategies for Eliminating Problem Foods

Once you've identified problem foods, consider the following strategies to remove or reduce them from your diet in a sustainable way:

1. *Start Gradually:* Instead of overhauling your diet overnight, start by reducing your intake of one or two trigger foods. For example, cut back on sugary snacks by swapping them for healthier alternatives, such as fresh fruits or unsweetened yogurt. Gradually, you can eliminate foods entirely without feeling deprived.

2. *Replace, Don't Remove:* Avoid leaving gaps in your meals when removing foods from your diet. Find healthier substitutes that offer similar flavors or textures. For example:
   - Replace white bread or pastries with whole-grain options like quinoa or oats.
   - Swap out sugary sodas for sparkling water infused with fresh lime or berries.
   - Use herbs and mild seasonings in place of spicy condiments like hot sauce or chili powder.

3. *Avoid "Hidden" Ingredients:* Problematic foods like sugar, refined carbs, and additives are often hidden in processed or pre-packaged items. Learn to read food labels carefully to avoid unintended consumption. Look for keywords like "added sugars," "high-fructose corn syrup," or "partially hydrogenated oils."

4. **Remove Temptation:** Keep your home stocked with healthy alternatives and remove items that are difficult to resist. For personal favorites like baked goods or salty snacks, reserve them for rare occasions and in smaller portions.

Experiment with Reintroduction

Eliminating certain foods entirely might not always be necessary or possible. Some people find that moderate consumption or only avoiding trigger foods during symptom flares is enough to manage their condition. Experimenting with reintroduction can help you determine your personal tolerance levels.

1. **Elimination Phase:** Begin by completely removing a suspected trigger food for two to three weeks. Observe whether your symptoms improve during this time.
2. **Reintroduction Phase:** Gradually add the eliminated food back into your diet in small amounts. For example, if you've been avoiding tomatoes due to their acidity, try incorporating them into one meal and monitor how you feel in the next 24-48 hours.
3. **Document Your Responses:** Track any symptoms that arise during the reintroduction phase in your food diary. If the symptoms return, you may need to avoid that food long-term or eat it only on rare occasions.
4. **Evaluate Moderation:** For foods like caffeine or alcohol, discover whether having smaller quantities at

certain times affects your symptoms less negatively. This approach gives you more flexibility while keeping symptoms manageable.

Monitor and Adjust Continuously

Even after eliminating problematic foods, it's essential to continue monitoring your diet and symptoms. Sjogren's Syndrome symptoms can change over time, meaning new triggers may emerge while others become less bothersome. Staying observant allows you to adapt as needed.

- *Update Your Food Diary:* Keep your food log active, noting any changes to symptoms, substitutions you've made, or new foods you've introduced.
- *Check for Seasonal Sensitivities:* During times of the year when dryness is more prevalent (e.g., winter), you may need to tighten your dietary restrictions to ease symptoms. Conversely, some foods may be easier to tolerate at other times.
- *Be Patient:* Reducing inflammation and observing improvements often take time. Give these dietary changes at least a few weeks to show meaningful results.

The Benefits of Personalized Adjustments

Eliminating or avoiding problematic foods might feel restrictive at first, but it paves the way for better symptom control and overall well-being. Personalizing this process ensures you're not depriving yourself unnecessarily while still reaping the benefits of improved comfort and energy.

- *Symptom Relief:* Most people find that eliminating triggers reduces flares, including dryness, pain, or energy crashes.
- *Improved Nutrition:* Removing sugary or processed options opens up space for nutrient-dense, healing foods that nourish your body.
- *Adaptable Eating Habits:* Over time, avoiding triggers becomes second nature, ensuring long-term compliance without the feeling of sacrifice.

Consult With Healthcare Professionals

Don't hesitate to involve healthcare providers in your dietary adjustments. They can help fine-tune your elimination plan, address concerns about nutritional balance, and suggest safe alternatives to potentially problematic foods.

- *Dietitians and Nutritionists:* These professionals can ensure you're not missing out on essential nutrients while avoiding trigger foods.
- *Rheumatologists:* Your specialist can advise how dietary changes complement your medical treatments and identify any interactions between certain foods and medications.

Avoiding or eliminating problematic foods is a powerful tool for managing Sjogren's Syndrome and enhancing your quality of life. By identifying your personal triggers, gradually reducing their role in your diet, and staying flexible with reintroduction strategies, you can create an eating pattern that supports your health and minimizes discomfort.

With time, patience, and guidance from professionals, this step equips you with valuable insights into how your body responds to food—giving you more control over your symptoms and allowing you to enjoy mealtimes with confidence.

Weekly Meal Plan

Ideally, making meal plans is a great way to help you transition from your regular meals to more diet-appropriate choices. Below is a sample meal plan made for a week that you can either follow or modify. The meals used below are based on the sample recipes provided in this guide.

Day 1

Breakfast: Breakfast Parfait

Snack: Healthy Green Smoothie

Lunch: Pecan and Maple Salmon

Dinner: Udon Salmon Soup

Day 2

Breakfast: Egg Salad with Avocado

Snack: A handful of raw almonds and walnuts for a mid-morning boost.

Lunch: Honey Chicken and Avocado Salad

Dinner: Celery Soup

Day 3

Breakfast: Sesame Cornmeal

Snack: Fresh berries with a drizzle of honey.

Lunch: Exotic Empanadas

Dinner: Orecchiette with Chickpeas and Broccoli Rabe

Day 4

Breakfast: Breakfast Parfait

Snack: A small bowl of diced cucumber topped with a dash of olive oil and pepper.

Lunch: Salmon Fry

Dinner: Mushroom Pastry

Day 5

Breakfast: Healthy Green Smoothie

Snack: Celery sticks with a small serving of almond butter.

Lunch: Pecan and Maple Salmon

Dinner: Vegetable Pasta in Avocado Sauce

Day 6

Breakfast: Egg Salad with Avocado

Snack: A handful of sunflower seeds and a cup of green tea.

Lunch: Honey Chicken and Avocado Salad

Dinner: Udon Salmon Soup

Day 7

Breakfast: Sesame Cornmeal

Snack: Greek yogurt topped with chia seeds and a pinch of cinnamon.

Lunch: Exotic Empanadas

Dinner: Orecchiette with Chickpeas and Broccoli Rabe

Consistency and variety are essential when managing Sjogren's Syndrome through diet. This meal plan introduces a mix of nourishing dishes that are rich in anti-inflammatory and antioxidant ingredients. Adjust portion sizes and substitute dishes as needed to fit your preferences and nutritional needs. Over time, these dietary habits can help reduce symptoms and improve your overall well-being.

Sample Recipes

Salmon Fry

Ingredients:

- salmon
- 1/2 tsp. smoked paprika
- 1/2 tsp. garlic powder

Instructions:

1. Coat the salmon with some garlic powder and paprika. Use other herbs if desired.
2. Place the salmon into the air fryer basket
3. Set the temperature of the Air Fryer to 400°F and cook for 10 minutes.
4. Serve and enjoy while hot.

No-Fuss Tuna Casserole

Ingredients:

- 1-5 oz. can tuna, drained
- 1 can cream of chicken soup, condensed
- 3 cups macaroni, cooked
- 1-1/2 cups fried onions
- 1 cup Cheddar cheese, shredded

Instructions:

1. Preheat the oven to 350°F.
2. Prepare a 9x13-inch baking dish. Use that to mix the macaroni, tuna, and soup. Top it with cheese.
3. Bake for 25 minutes or until the casserole is bubbly.
4. Sprinkle it with fried onions. Put back in the oven and leave for 5 more minutes.
5. Serve and enjoy while hot.

Pecan and Maple Salmon

Ingredients:

- 4 pcs. of 4 oz. salmon filet
- 1/2 tsp. onion powder
- 1/2 tsp. chipotle pepper powder
- 1 tbsp. apple cider vinegar
- 1 tsp. smoked paprika
- 1/2 cup pecans
- salt
- ground black pepper
- 3 tbsp. pure maple syrup

Instructions:

1. Lay salmon filets on a baking sheet.
2. Season them with salt and pepper.
3. In a food processor, pulse in pecans, vinegar, maple syrup, chipotle powder, paprika, and onion powder in a food processor. Continue doing so until the texture becomes crumbly.
4. Coat the top of the salmon filet with the pecan mixture.
5. Place the filet in the refrigerator without cover for about 2-3 hours.
6. Preheat the oven to 425°F.
7. Bake the salmon filet for about 12-14 minutes or until the filet flakes easily with a fork.

Celery Soup

Ingredients:

- 12-15 large stalks of celery, sliced half an inch
- 1 medium leek, thinly sliced
- 1 potato, peeled and cut into half-inch cubes
- 2 tbsp. butter
- 1 tbsp. fresh lime juice
- 6 cups water
- parsley, chopped
- salt

Instructions:

1. In a large saucepan, heat butter, followed by potato, celery, and leek over medium heat until the veggies start to soften.
2. Add the water to the saucepan and bring it to a boil.
3. Reduce heat to medium and simmer until vegetables are tender.
4. Puree soup in a blender or food processor until smooth.
5. Return soup to the pan; stir in lime juice and season with salt.
6. Serve warm and garnish with fresh parsley and celery leaves.

Egg Salad with Avocados

Ingredients:

- 3 medium-sized avocados
- 6 eggs, large and hard-boiled
- 1/3 red onion, medium size
- 3 celery ribs
- 4 tbsps. mayonnaise
- 2 tbsps. freshly squeezed lime juice
- 2 tsp. brown mustard
- 1/2 tsp. cumin powder
- 1 tsp. hot sauce
- salt
- pepper

Instructions:

1. Chop the eggs, celery, and onion.
2. Set aside the avocados, then combine the rest of the ingredients.
3. Slice the avocado in half to take out the pit.
4. Stuff the avocado by spooning the egg salad on its cage.
5. Serve and enjoy.

Honey Chicken and Avocado Salad

Ingredients:

- 4 chicken thighs, boneless
- 1/2 cup cherry tomatoes, halved
- 1/2 red onion, thinly sliced
- 1 head of romaine lettuce, chopped
- 2 avocados, chopped

Marinade:

- 1 tbsp. olive oil
- 1 tsp. salt
- 2 cloves garlic, minced
- 1 jalapeño pepper, minced
- 1/2 tsp. chili powder
- 1 tbsp. honey
- 4 tbsp. lime juice

Dressing:

- 1 tsp. salt
- 4 tbsp. olive oil
- 1/2 tsp. pepper
- 2 tbsp. honey
- 4 tbsp. lime juice

Instructions:

1. Combine all the chicken marinade ingredients in a container.
2. Add in the thighs and allow them to marinate for at least an hour.
3. Cook chicken in a cast-iron skillet on high heat for about 4 minutes on each side.
4. In a large salad bowl, put in avocados, lettuce, red onion, and tomatoes.
5. Slice or shred the chicken before adding it to the salad bowl.
6. In a separate bowl, combine the dressing ingredients and mix well.
7. While tossing the salad, add in the dressing.
8. Serve immediately.

Exotic Empanadas

Ingredients:

- 3 ox. lean ground beef
- 3 oz. mushrooms, chopped
- 1/4 cup onion, chopped finely
- 2 tsp. garlic, chopped finely
- 1/2 cup tomatoes, chopped
- 1/4 tsp. paprika
- 6 green olives, chopped
- 1/4 tsp. ground cumin
- 1/8 tsp. ground cinnamon
- 8 square gyoza wrappers
- 1 large egg, beaten
- 1 tbsp. olive oil

Instructions:

1. In a skillet, heat olive oil over medium-high heat.
2. Add in onions and garlic, sauté for about 2 minutes until fragrant.
3. Stir in ground beef and cook until browned.
4. Mix in mushrooms, tomatoes, paprika, cumin, and cinnamon.
5. Cook for an additional 5 minutes or until vegetables are softened.
6. Preheat oven to 375°F (190°C).

7. Lay out gyoza wrappers on a clean surface and spoon the filling into the center of each wrapper.

8. Brush the edges of the wrappers with beaten eggs before folding them over to form a triangle shape.

9. Press down firmly on the edges to seal.

10. Place empanadas on a baking sheet lined with parchment paper.

11. Brush the tops of the empanadas with beaten egg for a golden crust.

12. Bake for 15-20 minutes or until golden brown and crispy.

13. Serve hot and enjoy your exotic empanadas!

Crispy Pork Chop with Flavorful Brussels Sprouts

Ingredients:

- 8 oz. pork chop, bone-in and center-cut
- 6 oz. brussels sprouts
- 1/2 tsp. ground black pepper
- 1 tsp. olive oil
- 1 tsp. maple syrup
- 1 tsp. Dijon mustard
- cooking spray

Instructions:

1. In a bowl, put the pork chop and coat it lightly with cooking spray. Add half of the black pepper over it.
2. Take another bowl and add the oil along with maple syrup, dijon mustard, and remaining black pepper. Whisk them well.
3. In the mixture, add Brussels sprouts and toss it.
4. Place the marinated pork chop on one side of the air fryer basket. On the other side, place the coated sprouts.
5. Heat the air fryer to 400°F.
6. Place the basket and cook it until the pork turns golden brown.
7. After it turns golden, cook it for another 10 minutes to make it more tender.

Vegetable Pasta in Avocado Sauce

Ingredients:

- Zucchini Pasta
- 2 zucchini
- 3 cups red and yellow cherry tomatoes
- 4 oz. pasta
- Avocado Sauce
- 1/2 cup fresh parsley
- 1 tbsp. miso paste
- 1 garlic clove
- 1 avocado
- 1/4 cup olive oil
- 4 green onions
- 1/2 tsp. salt
- juice from 1 lemon
- ground pepper, to taste

Instructions:

1. To make the avocado sauce, use a blender to pulse all ingredients until smooth. Set aside.
2. In a large skillet over high heat, drizzle olive oil and cook cherry tomatoes until the skin loosens. Season with ground pepper and salt.

3. In the same skillet, add the zucchini and avocado sauce; toss to combine.
4. To serve, season with ground pepper and salt to taste; garnish with extra tomatoes.

Udon Salmon Soup

Ingredients:

- 8 oz. dried udon noodles, may also use ramen or soba, cooked and drained according to package instructions
- 1 clove garlic, smashed and peeled
- 4 oz. cremini mushrooms or button mushrooms, sliced thinly
- 2 scallions, sliced thinly
- 8 oz. salmon fillet, skinned and cut into 1-inch cubes
- 2 tbsp. white miso
- 1 cup boiling water
- 2 cups chicken or vegetable broth, homemade or store-bought, no salt added
- 1/2 tsp. seasoned rice vinegar
- 1 tsp. oyster sauce
- 1/4 tsp. toasted sesame oil

Instructions:

1. Boil a kettle of water.
2. Dissolve the miso in a cup of boiling water.
3. Pour the mixture through a fine-mesh strainer into a heavy saucepan or Dutch oven over medium heat.
4. Add broth, garlic, oyster sauce, and rice vinegar.
5. Once the mixture starts bubbling, reduce the heat to medium-low and cook for 5 minutes.

6. Stir in mushrooms and salmon. Cook for 15 minutes.
7. Remove the saucepan from the heat and stir in scallion, toasted sesame oil, and cooked udon noodles. Discard garlic.
8. Let sit for 3 to 5 minutes before serving.

Orecchiette with Chickpeas and Broccoli Rabe

Ingredients:

- 4 oz. whole wheat orecchiette
- 4 cloves garlic, minced
- 1/4 tsp. freshly ground pepper
- 1/2 bunch trimmed broccoli rabe, cut into 2-inch pieces
- 1/2 tsp. fresh rosemary, minced
- 3/4 cup chicken-flavored vegetarian broth
- 1 8-oz. can of chickpeas, drained and rinsed
- 2 tsp. all-purpose flour
- 2 tsp. red wine vinegar
- 1 tbsp. extra-virgin olive oil

Instructions:

1. Boil a large saucepan of salted water. Cook pasta in the salted water for 6 minutes.
2. Add broccoli rabe while stirring occasionally.
3. Cook the pasta and broccoli rabe for another 3 minutes before draining. Dry the pot.
4. Whisk flour and broth in a small bowl.
5. Sauté garlic and rosemary in a preheated pan over medium-high heat, stir constantly for a minute.

6. Whisk in the broth mixture and simmer. Stir constantly.
7. Add vinegar, chickpeas, pepper, salt, and the pasta mixture. Cook for a couple more minutes while stirring constantly.
8. Serve.

Sesame Cornmeal

Ingredients:

- 3/4 cup instant cornmeal
- 3 cups almond milk, an alternative for milk if you have acid reflux
- 1 tbsp. sesame seeds
- 3 tbsp. brown sugar
- 1 tsp. orange extract
- 1/2 tsp. vanilla extract
- salt, to taste

Instructions:

1. Pour almond milk into a saucepan. Bring to a boil.
2. Once boiling, add in the corn meal. Whisk well until a smooth consistency is achieved.
3. Add vanilla, orange extract, salt, and sugar to taste.
4. Garnish with sesame seeds.
5. Serve and enjoy.

Asian Fusion Mushroom Pastry

Ingredients:

- 100 g chestnut mushrooms, sliced into bite-size or strips
- 2 tbsp. coriander
- 35 g carrots, grated
- 1/2 tsp. Chinese 5 Spice Mix
- 2 shallots, diced
- 1 tsp. soy sauce
- 1 garlic clove, sliced and crushed
- 1 tbsp. breadcrumbs
- 1 chia egg or 1 tbsp. of ground chia seeds mixed in 1 tbsp. water
- 1/2 puff of pastry sheet
- olive oil
- unsalted butter
- salt
- white pepper

Instruction:

1. Preheat oven to 400°F (200°C). Line a baking sheet with parchment paper.
2. In a pan, heat olive oil and butter over medium-high heat. Add in the shallots and garlic. Cook until softened.

3. Add in the sliced mushrooms and grated carrots. Sauté for about 5 minutes or until the vegetables are tender.

4. Season with Chinese 5 spice mix, soy sauce, salt, and white pepper to taste.

5. Remove from heat and let it cool for a bit before adding in the chia egg or chia seed mixture.

6. Roll out puff pastry sheet on a floured surface into a large rectangle shape.

7. Spoon the mushroom mixture onto the pastry, leaving about 1-inch border around the edges.

8. Fold over the edges of the pastry and pinch to seal.

9. Place on a lined baking sheet and brush with beaten egg for a golden crust (optional).

10. Bake for 20-25 minutes or until the pastry is puffed and golden brown.

11. Sprinkle coriander on top before serving.

Breakfast Parfait

Ingredients:

- 7 tbsp. of thick, full-fat, live-culture yogurt, at ambient temperature
- 1/2 cup fresh, organic fruits except for bananas, at ambient temperature
- 3 tbsp. organic flax oil, chilled
- 2 tbsp. whole flaxseeds
- 1 tsp. raw honey, locally sourced
- ground cinnamon

Instructions:

1. Using a handheld coffee grinder, grind the flaxseeds.
2. Transfer the ground flaxseeds into a bowl.
3. Stir in the honey, and set aside.
4. Combine flax oil and yogurt in a blender.
5. Blend for about a minute, or until the texture has become creamy and the mixture has completely emulsified.
6. Pour the creamy mixture into the bowl with ground flaxseeds and honey.
7. Top with fruit, cinnamon, and nuts.

Healthy Green Smoothie

Ingredients:

- 1 cup fresh spinach
- 1/2 tsp. mint extract or to taste
- Optional: 1/4 tsp. peppermint liquid Stevia

Instructions:

1. Combine all ingredients in a blender or food processor.
2. Blend until smooth and creamy.
3. Serve immediately, or store in the refrigerator for up to 24 hours.
4. Optional: For a thicker consistency, add frozen fruit such as bananas or berries before blending.
5. Add more liquid, such as almond milk or coconut water, if needed to reach desired consistency.
6. Top with your favorite toppings, such as granola or chia seeds, for added nutrition and texture.
7. Enjoy this refreshing and nutritious drink any time of the day!

Conclusion

Thank you for taking the time to explore this comprehensive guide to Sjogren's Syndrome. By empowering yourself with knowledge, you've taken a crucial step toward better management and understanding of this complex condition. Whether you're navigating Sjogren's yourself or supporting a loved one, the insights you've gained can lead to meaningful improvements in daily life.

Living with Sjogren's Syndrome can sometimes feel overwhelming—but remember, you're not alone in this. The material covered here shows you that with the right tools, support, and strategies, it's possible to regain a sense of control and lead a fulfilling life. From understanding the science behind the condition to practical advice on managing symptoms, you now have a roadmap that can guide you.

One important takeaway is the value of a personalized approach. Every experience with Sjogren's is unique, so what works for one person might not work for another. That's why it's essential to listen to your body and adjust as needed. Whether it's dietary changes, mental health practices, or treatment plans, being patient while finding what suits you best is key. Small steps—like staying hydrated, leaning on anti-inflammatory foods, and prioritizing rest—can yield a big impact over time.

Caring for your emotional well-being is just as vital as managing physical symptoms. Chronic conditions can test your resilience, but practicing mindfulness, fostering connections with others, and seeking professional support can help you maintain balance. Don't forget to celebrate small victories—they matter. Even a day with slightly less fatigue or improved focus is a win on your health journey.

If you're supporting a friend or family member with Sjogren's, your efforts mean more than you might realize. By offering empathy, practical help, and encouragement, you're helping create a foundation for hope and healing. This guide provides practical tips and insights to strengthen your role, but never forget to care for your own well-being too. Supporting someone else works best when you first ensure your own health and energy reserves are cared for.

The beauty of learning about Sjogren's is that it opens doors—not just to understanding but also to action. With continued education and proactive choices, you or your loved one can significantly improve quality of life. Stay curious, and don't hesitate to tap into the many supportive communities, healthcare providers, and resources available. Having a solid support network can make all the difference.

As you move forward, think about how you can weave what you've learned into your daily life. Maybe it's trying a new recipe from the diet tips in this guide, reaching out to someone you've been meaning to connect with, or scheduling that overdue check-in with your doctor. Take it one step at a time, but keep stepping.

Thank you again for being part of this effort to understand and manage Sjogren's Syndrome. You've shown commitment, and that's already a victory.

Keep learning, keep adapting, and keep showing up for yourself or your loved one. You have what it takes to build a life that's not defined by limitations but rather by strength, self-care, and purpose. You're on the right path—and the future is brighter because of the steps you're taking today. Thank you for letting this guide be part of your journey.

FAQs

What is Sjogren's Syndrome, and what are its common symptoms?

Sjogren's Syndrome is a long-term autoimmune condition in which the immune system targets the glands responsible for producing moisture, causing dryness and inflammation. Common symptoms include dry eyes, dry mouth, fatigue, joint pain, and swollen salivary glands. Some individuals may also experience systemic issues affecting organs such as the lungs, kidneys, or nervous system.

How is Sjogren's Syndrome diagnosed?

Diagnosis typically involves a combination of medical history, physical exams, and specific tests. These may include blood tests to detect specific antibodies (like SSA/Ro and SSB/La), Schirmer's test to measure tear production, or a salivary gland biopsy to confirm inflammation. Since symptoms overlap with other conditions, an accurate diagnosis may take time and input from specialists like rheumatologists.

What treatment options are available for managing Sjogren's Syndrome?

While there's no cure, treatments focus on relieving symptoms and preventing complications. These may include artificial tears for dry eyes, saliva substitutes for dry mouth, medications like hydroxychloroquine for systemic symptoms, and immunosuppressants for severe cases. Lifestyle changes, such as a healthy diet and staying hydrated, also play an important role.

Can Sjogren's Syndrome affect pregnancy or breastfeeding?

Yes, Sjogren's may pose risks during pregnancy, such as preterm birth or conditions like neonatal lupus due to specific antibodies. Medications may need adjustment before and during pregnancy to ensure safety for both you and your baby. Breastfeeding can sometimes be challenging due to glandular dryness or medication concerns, so consulting with healthcare providers is crucial.

How can I manage fatigue and improve daily energy levels?

Managing fatigue starts with pacing yourself and prioritizing tasks. Create a balanced routine that includes rest periods, regular physical activity like yoga or walking, and a nutrient-rich diet. Flares can drain energy quickly, so having a "low-energy" plan in place—such as simple tasks or meals—can be helpful. Don't hesitate to lean on your support network for assistance with daily activities.

What lifestyle adjustments can help manage symptoms of Sjogren's Syndrome?

Simple adjustments can make a significant difference, such as using a humidifier at home, wearing sunglasses to protect your eyes, drinking water frequently, and avoiding alcohol or caffeine that worsens dryness. Anti-inflammatory foods and stress management practices, like mindfulness or meditation, can help reduce symptom severity.

Where can I find support and resources to cope with Sjogren's Syndrome?

Support is available through national organizations, such as the Sjogren's Foundation, which offers education, forums, and connect groups. Online communities and local support groups can also provide emotional encouragement and practical advice. Speaking with counselors or therapists who specialize in chronic illness can further aid mental well-being and resilience.

References and Helpful Links

Ghafoor, M. (2011). Sjögren's Before Sjögren: Did Henrik Sjögren (1899–1986) really discover Sjögren's disease? Journal of Maxillofacial and Oral Surgery, 11(3), 373–374. https://doi.org/10.1007/s12663-011-0303-0

Laliberte, M. (2024, July 29). Sjögren's symptoms: 11 clues you might be ignoring. CreakyJoints. https://creakyjoints.org/living-with-arthritis/symptoms/sjogrens-syndrome-symptoms/

Sjögren's Foundation, Inc. (2021, January 13). Nutrition to improve symptoms of Sjögren's. Sjögren's Foundation. https://sjogrens.org/blog/2021/nutrition-to-improve-symptoms-of-sjogrens

News-Medical. (2019, May 1). Sjogren's Syndrome related disorders. https://www.news-medical.net/health/Sjogrens-Syndrome-Related-Disorders.aspx

Sjogren syndrome: MedlinePlus Medical Encyclopedia. (n.d.). https://medlineplus.gov/ency/article/000456.htm#:~:text=Sj%C3%B6gren%20syndrome%20is%20an%20autoimmune,including%20the%20kidneys%20and%20lungs.

Pregnancy and Sjögren's. (n.d.). Sjögren's Foundation. https://sjogrens.org/living-with-sjogrens/pregnancy-and-sjogrens

Sjögren's Disease. (n.d.).
https://rheumatology.org/patients/sjogrens-disease

What foods are good and bad for Sjogren's syndrome? (2021, February 26). MedicineNet.
https://www.medicinenet.com/what_foods_are_good_and_bad_for_sjogr ens_syndrome/article.htm

www.ingramcontent.com/pod-product-compliance
Lightning Source LLC
LaVergne TN
LVHW020224080925
820513LV00033B/1326